TAKE JOY IN GROWING OLD, DAGNABBIT!

Susan
To Bob
Keep on taking
joy in life!
Blessings!
Joe Hall

JOE DONALD HALL

outskirtspress

DENVER, COLORADO

INTRODUCTION

Joy is a special treasure intended for all of us, but it keeps on escaping from most of us. In fact, some never find it. Others seem to have captured **joy**, and it has become their way of life.

I became intrigued with the question— Why? What makes the difference in a person of **joy** and one without **joy**? The difference is especially pronounced as people age. In observing and talking to men and women that are aging it seemed to me that the difference is truly striking.

So I set about to discover and convey the differences.

I found there are some threads that are

common to the aging who possess and are sharing their **joy**. I have tried to describe these common threads.

I have titled the book *Take Joy in Growing Old, Dagnabbit!* I use the word **take** because I think **joy** is there for the taking. It turns out to be a choice, or series of choices. All of us **can** have **joy**. Once you have **joy**, it's more about being than doing—**joy** becomes who you are.

I write to anyone who is striving to live with **joy**, but especially to those striving while aging. Life itself is difficult, especially as we age. For me, **joy** is the game changer. Taking **joy** in life could be the game changer for you too!

God bless you for your efforts toward **joy**.

Perhaps this little book will help, **dagnabbit!**

This book is dedicated to

Barbara Ellen Hall

1933-2012

My wife of 58 years, the inspiration for this work, and the most **joyful** person I have ever known

ACKNOWLEDGMENTS

The writing of this book took place over a 3-year period. I received support, guidance, suggestions, and counsel from many friends, neighbors, family, reviewers, retirement center residents, writers, and folks that were intrigued with the subject of **joy**. To attempt to list them all would be futile, but it is safe to say that there would be no "Dagnabbit" book without their help and support.

The three I would mention by name are my granddaughters, Bailey, Paige, and Andrea. All in their 20s, they were my technical and advisory team. From typing to revising, corrections to transmitting, editing to publishing, and just encouraging me, these three beautiful women carried the load and delivered the product.

Whether named or not—THANK YOU!

TABLE OF CONTENTS

EDGAR AND LEROY: THE BEGINNING

═══════════

"Edgar, what makes you so all fired joyful all the time?" Leroy asked as the two sat in easy chairs at the retirement center. The two often spend time together at the center where they now live, since both are widowed, and they seem to enjoy each other's company most of the time.

"What in the cat hair are you talking about, Leroy?" asked Edgar.

Leroy replied, "I'm talking about you being joyful. I just can't figure it out. Look, I've been thinking," Leroy continued, "we have a lot of similar things in our lives, but you seem to live and cherish each day, while I wake up sorry that I didn't die during the night. I mean, both our wives have passed on, we're both in our 70s, we both have kids and grandkids that don't always make good choices in life, neither of us are rich but are managing to pay our bills, both of us are in tolerable health, both of us are lonely at times, and lots of other things. But I can hardly stand my life, while you seem to really take joy in life every day. Edgar, you're the best friend I've got, but it's beginning to bug me. I just can't understand how the two of us can be so similar, almost identical, yet our joy in life is, well, almost totally opposite."

"Well," Edgar mused as he stroked his scruffy gray beard, "not sure I've got all the answers, but let me give it a shot. First off, you sure as heck don't have to be joyful;

in fact, most of the folks I know at our age don't have much real joy, or if they do, it sure doesn't show!"

Edgar continued. "Another thing to keep in mind is that joy and happiness are not synonymous! They are kin but not the same. Happiness is more external, or controlled by events going on in or around our lives, while joy is more internal. Happiness seems to be fleeting while joy sticks around. Happiness, seems to me, is mostly man-made, while joy, I think, is more God-driven. I'm not saying you need to get all 'churchy' and stuff, but I believe I wouldn't have much joy if I didn't have God in my life. At least for me, it sure helps to know God is on my side!"

"You know, Leroy, this is something **you** can do! You are capable and qualified to **take joy** in your life. You see, it turns out to be a choice, or series of choices that purposefully set the direction for joy." Leroy tried to interrupt, but Edgar stopped him. "Yep, I know **exactly** how old you are... You're not too old! **You can** do this!"

Edgar continued. "What are these choices and directions that allow us to take joy in our lives? I would like for you to walk through this short book with me, *Take Joy in Growing Old, Dagnabbit!* The book simply traces some of the threads that seem to be consistent in older folks that have somehow managed to find **joy** in life at an advanced age. I think it would be worth your time."

"OK, then," replied Leroy, "I'm gonna go through the dumb book with you, but I'm not promising to like it, and sure as heck not promising to take joy!

Edgar chuckled and said, "Let's get on with it, **dagnabbit**!"

CHAPTER 1:
WHAT IS THIS JOY?

═══════════════

"Old is when...everything hurts and what doesn't hurt, doesn't work."

"Seems to me a man with no fear can't have any love in his life, and with no love there is no **joy**...of course, I could be wrong," said King Arthur to Lancelot in the movie *First Knight*.

Lancelot had just told King Arthur that he had no fear and that is the reason he was so successful in battle. The king, after encouraging Lancelot to stay in Camelot, then mused the question…"Without love, where is the **joy**?"

The king said he could be wrong—but I don't think so. I think he nailed it! As Sherwood Wirt puts it, "You can have love without **joy**, but you can't have joy without love."

Maybe **joy** is a state of being—a state some have found, but most of us have not. The irony is that we haven't found it because we're seeking it for ourselves. People who have found **joy** have done so by giving it to someone else. Once the joyful discover this treasure, they just keep on giving, keep on loving, and keep on being **joyful**.

Now let's be clear, we're not talking about **joy** in the afterlife. That's a given—there **will** be **joy** in heaven! What we are talking about is **joy** in this life, here, and now. And we are talking about joy in older folks. That's right! As we age we should be the most joyful people on the planet. After all, as we age we've mostly figured out how this life is going to play out. We know who our real friends are, have an understanding of who God is, know what our purpose in life is, and perhaps most importantly, we're ALMOST HOME.

Now, I'm blessed that in my old age I have a great family and I still have friends alive who live close. I have some older friends who clearly have joy, and I have some older friends who clearly don't. Two aging individuals with similar issues and challenges can have opposite attitudes about life. Go figure. Both are in retirement, both are lonely and do not receive many visitors, both have limited but adequate financial resources, both are in failing health and yet, one is joyful and one is not. WHY?

I'm just a Texas Aggie so how in the "cat

hair" would I know? I've just observed and interviewed aging folks, so the best I can come up with are common threads that seem to run through the joyful aging camp. The threads are:

THE JOYFULLY AGING, for the most part, did not get that way overnight. Generally the old guy full of joy was a young guy full of joy and the old grump was likely at one time a young grump. I'm not saying one can't change. Of course, someone can change! But my observation has been that most of my older friends are pretty much how they were in their younger lives, only more pronounced—one way or the other. Those who "get it" and discover real joy in their lives tend not only to keep it, but the joy grows with the years. In fact, they seem to become **"joy spreaders."** The grumps, well, what can I say? They just get grumpier. So, a word here to those not yet old, but hoping to get there someday—start now! Start taking joy in life by bringing joy to others. Then old age, when it comes, will be a blessing for you and those around you. The earlier in life we take joy in life, the better.

THE JOYFULLY AGING has figured out how to cope with or even ignore adversity. We all have things going wrong in our lives, and it gets worse as we age. Some of those close to us die. Our children and grand-children get caught up in difficulties we never could imagine. Our health is failing, or we've lost our independence, or people no longer seem to care about us, and… well, you get it. Life's adversities don't go away as we age, they just keep growing. Those filled with joy seem to cope with adversity, smile, and keep on truckin'.

THE JOYFULLY AGING has figured out

how to live one day at a time. The older we get the less we can count on even having another day, much less on how the future days are going to go. So the focus of people aging joyfully is today. The joyful tend to not look too far ahead. So, live joyfully today, bring joy to someone today, love today, and hopefully, tomorrow, you'll do it all over again. But, hey, let's worry about that tomorrow. If we need to improve a relationship or encourage someone or call an old friend, it's not "I need to do that someday." Do it today!

THE JOYFULLY AGING, without exception in my experience, do not spend much time or energy thinking about themselves. They are forever focused on others and how they might bring some joy into their lives! Perhaps it goes deeper than the fact that it is what these joyfully aging people **do**—it is who they **are**. It is not so much about doing, it is more about being! It is who you are—a joyful person—or not. Seems like for some it has become so much a part of them they don't even need to consciously turn from themselves to others; it's just what they do.

I know for me this is an uphill battle as I get **really** old. My natural tendency is to think about myself—and only me. Every time I find myself down in the dumps I've discovered it's because I'm focused on me. I seem to never get down when my concern, prayers, and effort are centered on others.

THE JOYFULLY AGING has managed to retain their self-respect. All of us older folk share in common overriding, nagging, and increasing facts of life—we're just not the same man or woman we once were! You name it, from athletics to penmanship to technology, we've gone downhill. Some let this phenomenon drag their whole lives down. They spiral downward with self-pity, have an ever-increasing downcast look, and seem to take it out on others. Linda Ronstadt captured it in a song she recorded years ago titled "Poor, Poor, Pitiful Me." The joyful seem to take aging in stride and get on with life. Seems to me a lot of the things they're not good at anymore are replaced by adding the "fruit of the Spirit," especially love, joy, and peace.

THE JOYFULLY AGING all have a purpose. Having purpose is something that works for them. It may not be as lofty as "world peace," but is something that gives them a reason to begin each day and begin it with joy.

THE JOYFULLY AGING have discovered the joy in lasting, continuing, quality relationships. They cherish them and do their part in making them better.

THE JOYFULLY AGING have discovered the distinctive **joy** that comes from being in the Lord. Although I strongly favor church attendance, that alone is not "being in the Lord." Just sitting in a church building every Sunday for years will no more make you a joyful person than sitting in a garage will make you a Toyota! Most people filled with joy understand and practice what Jesus said about living life in the "Sermon on the Mount," which is the greatest commandment: "To love God with all your heart and love your neighbors as yourself." King Arthur was right—Without love there is just no joy!

⋙〰⋘

Surely there's something to be gained by

examining these threads of the joyful, and we'll explore them together as we proceed through this book.

Here's the thing: God is joy, Jesus is joy, and it was intended that we have joy. Jesus came to earth so that we might have joy. But some of us have just missed the boat. It's not too late. We **can** change! We **can** be what God intended, even in old age. No, **especially** in old age! Take joy in growing old, **dagnabbit!**

CHAPTER 2:
GROWING OLD

A funny thing happened on the way to old age. I realized I could get old and still have **joy**!

As Jonathon Swift said, "Everyone wants to live long, but no one wants to be old." There is so much dread of being old, but it can be a time of happiness, fulfillment, and **joy**!

Sure, there are a lot of hurdles as we age. For example:

- Some friends have gone on, some just lost interest.

- Kids and grandkids have other interests; perhaps they don't value my "wisdom."

- Health is not at all what it used to be.

- I have regrets about some aspects of the life I've lived.

- On the other hand, we've also got some real advantages:

- Learning to cherish each and every day.

- We can live to bring **joy** into someone's life, not just exist for today.

- We can decide to live joyously regardless of what goes on outside of us and use our internal strength to think of others and serve others.

After all, we're ALMOST HOME, and I

want to do more than "not fumble in the red zone." For all I know, this is exactly the time that God has allowed me to live for. This is the time I might influence others or contribute to a solution or make a difference in someone's life. I might still MATTER!

The question is: Do we enter old age with joy? The answer is closely aligned with the answer to the question posed by a friend, "Should it make a difference how we view and deal with the 'golden years' whether we are a Christian or not?"

S. D. Gordon said, "Joy is distinctly a Christian word and a Christian thing." I think the whole notion of joy is God's idea! God created us to have joy, but joy in Him. Jesus had joy and spread it. The real tragedy is when a person tries to serve God faithfully all of their lives, but they still never feel joy or peace. They go about life so serious, sad, and even gloomy, and then no one wants what they've got! After all, as William Barclay says, "A gloomy Christian is a contradiction in terms!"

As another friend recently shared with me, "Live each day at work as though it were your first, live each day at home as though it were your last." For those of us in the aging department, today may actually be our last so we should live accordingly. This may be the last day for me to spread joy, so I need to get at it.

———⚬———

I think Albert Einstein said it best, "Never grow old, no matter how long you live." Well, I've lived long, and I'm trying not to allow myself to become old. Let's just say things are different now. It's now my doctor who tells me to slow down rather than the police. Most of the stuff I've read on aging has been written by younger authors still in their 30s and 40s. It's not that their thoughts and counsel are not valid; it's just that they've not been old yet. It's not that they are ignorant; it's just that they think they know so much, and it may not work for some of us.

I have asked myself why I would want to undertake the chore of writing this book. The answer is that if I'm going to help even a few senior folks sort things out in their older years, I sort of need to do it while I'm still alive! When a friend of Oliver Wendell Holmes asked him why he had taken up the study of Greek at age 94, his response was, "Well, my good sir, it's now or never." For some of us growing old, we seem to be reluctant, even frightened, as we embark on any new challenge. This might be the very reason we're still here, to contribute information in a caring way to our fellow senior citizens that could possibly make a difference in their lives. The Christian author Max Lucado wrote, "God's oldest have always been among his choicest."

At one time I liked the phrase "Don't fumble in the red zone" to describe our approach to old age. It is a football term that means don't make a mistake once you get inside the 20-yard line. In other words, don't mess up near the goal line. I once thought that made sense; just play it safe as you get old. I've changed my mind. Now I don't think it's the right direction to play it "safe." We should take chances and take on new challenges! God doesn't want us to quit before the end, and for cryin' out loud, don't die before you're dead! The irony is that by playing it safe, not reaching out to help, not establishing that new relationship or making an existing relationship better, or just taking the safe route, we might indeed fumble in the "red zone" since we've stopped doing what God has planned for us here.

—⟨⟩—

The difference in living life with or without joy is striking, and it is clear. I have seen this difference personally with two friends. One maintains a joyful approach to life while the other seems to be in a negative death spiral on the happiness scale. Both have had serious surgeries, and both are plagued with their respective families pretty much deserting them in their old age.

From one all I ever hear are negative statements about how bad things are. He always complains about his health. No one has ever had it this bad. He says his kids and grandkids not only don't visit him, but they no longer even care about his views—on anything. He believes they are out to get what's left of his money and will likely bury him in a cheap pine box. Oh, and he seldom smiles and never, ever laughs.

On the other hand, the other friend smiles a lot and has the best laugh I've ever heard. He talks positively about his family. He doesn't complain that they never visit him, but he points out the good works that they do and their successes at work or school. He makes light of his physical problems and says, "It will be better someday" and "a lot of folks have it worse than me."

Guess which one I'd rather be with? I look forward to being with the joyful friend and dread my time spent with the other. I'm not exactly sure why these two friends have almost exactly the same situation in their lives but are miles apart in their approach to life. It seems that while one is always thinking about himself the other is focused on others, including me. The result, as far as I can tell, is that one takes joy in life, **even in growing old**, while the other simply does not.

Now don't get me wrong. I think it's hard to take joy in life as life's conditions deteriorate. When one has a son on death row in the penitentiary, or has a spouse with Alzheimer's, or is on death's doorstep due to cancer, well, it's just harder not to think of yourself. But this one thing I'm pretty sure of. If I spend the bulk of my time thinking about all the negative things that adversely affect me, then I'm a "no-hoper" for living a joyous, happy life in my sunset years!

Another thing about my joyful friend is he seems to have a distinct joy in being in the Lord. In fact, that seems to be a common thread in the happy and joyous older folks—I know that they have joy in their faith. It seems like when you think about it, God did not create us to be sour and miserable. Jesus seemed to have joy, and said that He came to earth so that we might have joy. Yet many of us churchgoers have managed to turn church (and religion, in general) into an all-too-serious, down-in-the mouth, seldom joyful experience. I don't think God is too happy about that. God is in heaven waiting for us with a smile on His face, and He is ticked, I believe, that we're not smiling enough. I intend to ask God if I'm right about that when I get to heaven!

Also, it seems like it is possible to lose your joy. Some believers apparently had already started to "lose it" soon after Jesus left this earth. We can tell this due to the Apostle Paul asking the Galatians, "What has happened to all your joy?"

I asked Laverne, a 96-year-old retired schoolteacher about this notion. She said to me, "The real joy comes from being in the Lord and loving Him. It is only when we love God that He gives us joy. It's definitely a distinctive joy."

We have learned that we can have love without joy, but that we cannot have joy without love. As for LaVerne, she now takes joy in seeing a deer outside the window of her assisted living apartment, and the snowfall, and being contacted by a former student. She tries every day to "reach out to someone in a way that might cause them to seek God."

Jesus was a man of joy. While talking to

the guys closest to Him about remaining faithful and bearing fruit He said, "I have told you these things so that MY **JOY** MAY BE IN YOU AND THAT YOUR **JOY** MAY BE COMPLETE." In my mind, there is no question that God intends for us to be full of joy!

———

Now a word about my hearing aids. Yes, my hearing aids! You see, I've learned something that needs sharing. It's not that I've learned about hearing aid technology, frequencies, battery life, costs, or best brands. What I have learned is that all this doesn't help until you...

1) TURN THE HEARING AIDS ON

and

2) PUT THEM IN YOUR EARS! AMAZING!

All the knowledge and expertise in the world doesn't amount to a "hill of beans" unless you actually put them to use.

WOW! What a concept! There's got to be a lesson here someplace. Perhaps, like hearing aids, it's that some of us have let joy become an intellectual concept, but we've forgotten that it only works when you put it into practice. It's only when we actually realize that God's plan is for us to be joyful, to allow us individually to become a person of joy, and to become a "**joy spreader**," that the whole concept really works. That's so simple it's scary, but then I like simple, and I sort of think God does too!

TAKE JOY IN GROWING OLD, DAGNABBIT!

So, what about being old? You think God had us old people in mind when He had the stuff in the Bible written about joy?

"Surely you jest, God," we might say. "Have you any idea the troubles I've got? Perhaps, God, you just don't understand old age. Oh, never mind, I suppose you do!"

One day at lunch a friend asked me, "What is old?" I remembered these:

OLD IS WHEN…Your children begin to look middle-aged.

OLD IS WHEN…Every conversation with someone in your age group includes at least one medical report.

And finally,

OLD IS WHEN…Former classmates are so gray, wrinkled, and bald they don't recognize you.

We like to joke about being old, and that's good since as someone said, "If you don't laugh at trouble you won't have anything to laugh at when you are old." Not sure what age that is when everyone starts to feel old, but for me, I think it was 75. Reaching the three-quarter century mark made me realize I still had time to do some good, but I needed to get crackin'. Surely at some age one should acknowledge—yep, I'm old! It's your perspective on being old that matters. If you view it like some, that most old folks are mean-spirited, cantankerous, sick, isolated, and useless, then, of course, you dread the thought of becoming old. The other side is those that are able to see the joyous side of aging, or **take joy in growing old**, somehow manage to find within themselves what God intended…an inner peace, love, and joy. Old is not bad. In fact, old is good if we let it be.

As far as still being able to accomplish significant achievements in older age, it's a no-brainer. Just look at the accomplishments of older people like Benjamin Franklin or Winston Churchill or J. C. Penny, and Dr. Lillien Martin. Numerous others have shown time after time that old age does not equate to useless...unless we let it!

Batsell Barrett Baxter, a Christian minister, wrote an article titled "Conquering Life's Problems." He suggested the following ideas to better cope with old age.

- Consider life a sowing and reaping process.

- Develop a proper attitude toward service.

- Retain your self-respect during older years.

- Listen to other people, rather than giving advice which they may not want.

- Accept physical and mental limitations gracefully.

- Communicate with other people.

- Place high value on time.

- Cultivate a sense of humor that will allow you to enjoy laughing with others.

- Grow spiritually.

As Einstein said, "Never grow old, no matter how long you live"—(**dagnabbit!**)

CHAPTER 3:
RELATIONSHIPS
(A cherished treasure!)

OLD IS WHEN…"Getting lucky" means you find your car in the parking lot.

Bobby, John, and William were my buddies when I was a teenager. There was nothing we wouldn't try—no fight we would shy away from—no game we couldn't win—as long as we were together. We were quick to belittle each other, but even quicker to defend each other. We gave each other such a hard time that we never stopped to realize what we really had. I now realize that close friends are tough to come by, and for some people, having close friendships never happens at all. Bobby, John, William, and I never gave any thought to cherishing and preserving our friendship. Shoot, we probably couldn't even spell "cherish"!

Well, okay, but we were just kids, you say, but what about those of us who are now aging? We can easily forgive a kid for not realizing the value of friendships and family, but you'd think by the time we're old we'd know better. You'd think we might have learned by now how to tell our friends and family what they mean to us. You'd think we would've learned to cherish and take **joy** in friends and family—**dagnabbit!** Many of us still act like kids when it comes to true relationships. Whether with our mates, our grandkids, or friends of many years, we just roll on, year by year, assuming that relationships just happen, and they will last forever.

With aging, quality, lasting relationships are as important as anything when it comes to living a joyful, meaningful life. Getting old is no picnic, but without real relationships it's almost a "no-hoper," a term my teenage buddies used to call each other. With friends and family at your side, you can approach each new dawn with a renewed spirit, and each night with a sense of fulfillment. You can experience the joy of being loved, and more importantly, know the joy of loving, or giving love.

I've been blessed in this life with many close friends and family. They are not just casual acquaintances, but real, intimate relationships. Those where you can be the real you, warts and all, and they love you anyway. The names of those close to me are no longer Bobby, John, and William, but I share a current bond with my friends just as strong. In fact, the bonds are tighter.

Our relationships are rich! These relationships made me realize that I am a rich man in every way that matters.

I recently found a way to tell three of my closest friends what they mean to me. It was on the first tee of the golf course—and you know what? It wasn't that hard to do! I found that they felt the same way, but had also experienced difficulty in telling me. Isn't it amazing? That four old guys in old age discovered what we should have figured out many years ago—**to cherish your loved ones and tell them you love them, and then do your part in making those relationships stronger.**

Maintaining quality, lasting relationships in old age requires some special effort, and it is well worth the work. It seems to me that quality relationships rank right up there, near the top, in importance as we

age if we want to joyfully age. Keeping relationships can get difficult with age. Some
of the reasons we have problems with relationships as we age are:

- Our friends die! The longer we live,
  the more funerals we'll attend for
  friends and family. As we age, these
  deaths and funerals can become a
  real problem. I know some who feel
  all alone because all of their friends
  have just "died off."

- Mobility is an increasing dilemma.
  We may become unable to move
  around independently, and the logis-
  tics of getting together with friends
  and family becomes difficult. When
  neither you nor your friends can drive
  any longer, it is just harder! Well,
  how about texting each other? You've
  gotta be kidding!

- Change is hard. We all change with age. Sometimes the erosion of time just makes it difficult to remain close. Family members also change. If I'm still loving a grandchild and remembering her as she was as a little girl and she's now grown up and married with children of her own, there's little chance for a continual relationship. It's important to treat grown grandchildren with respect and love. Cherish them as adults to keep a loving, quality relationship.

Let's concentrate on bringing some focus to our relationships. Stop taking relationships for granted and start working to make them even better. If you need help on bringing focus to your relationships, here are a few steps to begin with:

- REALIZE what you've got. Just stop

for a moment and focus on the individual and count your blessings.

- CHERISH the relationship. Just imagine how much you would miss them if the relationship were gone.

- FORGIVE! Not all your friends and family are perfect. Well, actually, none of them are perfect, right? But most of us have figured out that we're not either. If you're harboring a grudge or resentment or anger over something a dear one has done or failed to do—get over it! Your relationship will never be all that it can be until you completely forgive! I'm talking forgiveness by name, by the specific act and not the old, "I'll forgive—but I'll not forget" syndrome. You may or may not even need to tell the individual that you forgive them, just do it—NOW!

- LOVE them, just love them!

- TELL them you love them and tell them you cherish them. Share what they mean to you. And here's a radical idea: TELL THEM WHILE YOU ARE BOTH STILL ALIVE!

Here's the thing—if the closest relationships we have in life are not bringing us joy, then something needs to improve. God gave us one another for a reason, and I believe a large part of that reason is to bring us joy. To joyfully age, it is critical to have quality relationships. Do your part. It's worth it, **dagnabbit!**

CHAPTER 4:
IT'S NOT ABOUT ME
(At least not ALL about me!)

═══════════════

OLD IS WHEN…An "all-nighter" means not going to the bathroom the entire night.

One of my first jobs as a young teen was working as a bus boy in the Sara Ann Café in East Dallas, Texas. It was a small place where the food was served from a steam table. It was more "blue collar" than fine dining, but blue collar was the way of life in my neighborhood. I cleaned the tables, set up for the next customer, sometimes re-filled coffee cups, sometimes washed dishes. The Sara Ann was located just across the alley from a large church, and on Sunday mornings, we were usually cram packed. Many of the men at that time dropped off their families for Sunday school, then headed across the alley to the café for coffee and cigarettes and some serious "bull shooting" with their buddies.

One of these Sunday mornings I got my first glimpse of my "it's all about me" side. One of the tables had men who were especially demanding and rude. Since I was a kid, it was easy for them to harass me and give me a hard time. After a little while, I went to see the café owner, who, as usual, was manning the steam table. The owner said to do whatever I wanted or needed to, since the "church" never spent any money in the Sara Ann anyway. I marched right over to that table and asked them to leave—I threw them out. They checked with the owner, and he backed me up. I still remember his statement, "Whatever Joe says." I was so pleased, so proud, so pumped up. "Just look at me, I actually threw some grown-ups out!"

Later that day, while walking home from work, it dawned on me why I was so happy about the experience. It was because it had been all about me, my hurt feelings when they yelled at me, and my revenge on all the evildoers. It occurred to me on the lonely walk home that I didn't give a thought about the guys at the table. How ironic is that? I was a "server" but not the least bit interested in actually serving. I didn't spend a single moment thinking about whether their gripes had merit or if their misbehavior was well-founded. Sure, they were wrong—but so was I. I threw them out because I was empowered to do so, but more important, because it made me feel good. I got 'em, **dagnabbit!**

Well, I wasn't as proud on the walk home, and as I age I'm still not proud when my actions, or lack of actions, are all about me. As I think about the times when I allow myself to get down in the dumps, guess what? It's always when I'm thinking about myself. I'm just never down when I'm focused on others and how to serve them.

In the interviews and discussions I've had with aging folks one thing is clear: Those aging joyfully have developed the trait of focusing on others, not themselves!

In the seventeenth century, Blaise Pascal set forth the premise that all of life is about searching for happiness. He said, "All human beings seek happiness...It is the motive of every action of every human being, even those who hang themselves. Yet without faith no one ever reaches the goal of happiness toward which we all aspire." He further said that, "We should be convinced, based on evidence from the beginning of time, of our inability to reach the good life by our own efforts." Perhaps this is our first clue—that seeking happiness (and joy) for ourselves and by ourselves has never worked, and never will.

So, I think my joyfully aging friends are on to something. They have figured out how to arrive at the place in their lives where their thoughts are on others, not themselves. Of course, some of their thoughts are about themselves and always will be, but the focus of their lives is on others. That's why each day the joyfully aging wake up thinking, "Which old friend do I need to call? How can I encourage a grandchild? How can I reach out to someone, or improve a relationship? TODAY!"

I'm not sure Pascal was right when he

said that every human action is about our own happiness, but his conclusion helps lead us in the right direction, especially as it relates to JOY. The individual attains joy by giving it away. We can't earn joy; we can only give it to someone else.

I like my friend Dr. Jack Wasinger's example of the difference between happiness and joy. He says if a guy on the street corner is handing out one hundred dollar bills, everyone that gets one is happy, but the only one with joy is the guy giving them out.

Perhaps this "not about me" notion is worth some prayerful consideration. We should make a daily commitment to make each day about others, **dagnabbit!**

CHAPTER 5:
SELF-RESPECT
(No longer a spiker!)

═══════════════

OLD IS WHEN...You are cautioned to slow down by your doctor instead of the police.

Several years ago, I got into a volleyball game at the park with some friends. When it came my time to move to the front line I relished the first opportunity to spike the ball—as I've done many times over the years. My chance came, a beautiful setup, I jumped, made a great swing—and my spike went right into the middle of the net! Several other chances came my way with similar results. As it turns out, my "jump" was perhaps 3 inches off the ground and my "great swing" was, well—not! I finally said to my teammates, "I think I should be a setter." I switched and actually did quite well setting the ball for others to spike. I just was not what I used to be on the volleyball court. I was no longer a "spiker"!

The aging process brings most of us to a realization that we're just not what we used to be. For some, unfortunately, that equates to being worthless and leads to a serious loss of self-respect.

It is tough to see the diminishment of what you've been good at all your life. I know as a man, whether I'll admit it or not, that I'm concerned parts of me that were present in my young and productive years are, for the most part, behind me. It's not just the loss of my athletic ability I've been concerned about. As we old guys are inclined to say, "The older we get, the better we used to be!" After all, I used to earn a living, have people working for me, was a good public speaker, had children at home that sometimes listened to me, mowed my own yard, and well…You get the idea. It was a little shocking to discover that from the boardroom to the bedroom, I'm just not the same man I used to be. I would guess women have the same aging discouragements, plus one added concern…Their looks are changing. Although I believe older women are still beautiful, I have learned from discussions I've had that many women believe because they have lost their good looks that they have also lost some self-respect.

The problem is that in losing self-respect we, in fact, do become a different person. When we no longer see ourselves as a person of worth, a contributor to life with purpose in our lives, we retreat into the world within. We become increasingly lonely, isolated, feel sorry for ourselves, and are downright miserable to be around. We have entered the death spiral of self-pity, from which few recover.

When I thought this out, I needed to ask the tough question—am I better at anything than I used to be? For the answer I looked to what God said He wanted us to get better at—what He called the "fruits of the Spirit" (Galatians 5:22–23). They are: love, joy, peace, patience, kindness, goodness, faithfulness, gentleness, and self-control. I wondered how I was doing in these nine areas of life. So I asked myself, are you better, worse, or about the same as you were, say, 30 years ago? You know what, **dagnabbit**…I'm better in all (well, actually there's one where I'm about the same) of them! But here's the thing…I'm actually closer to what God wants me to be than when I was a spiker and a speaker. It is exciting for me to realize that I'm actually getting closer to the person God desires. I am, in every way that matters, a very rich man.

God had the writer call them "fruit." Perhaps He had it figured out that some of His folks like me might take awhile to grow in their "fruit." It could be that some of us need the successes and failures of a long life to understand what's important to God and what should really matter to us.

It's interesting that joy is listed second, right behind love. Some have said, "You can have love without joy, but you can't have joy without love." I'm inclined to agree with that. In fact, it seems to me that the first three (love, joy, and peace) are so intertwined that they are inseparable. It is only in loving as God wants us to love that we are able to take joy in life, and that gives us peace. When you think about it—amazing!

So, what about your volleyball game of life? Is it the way you thought it would be or not even close to the peak performance you gave? So what! Here's the deal. Everyone who is aging faces these facts. Sooner or later, we all must come to grips with the notion that our young and productive years are, for the most part, behind us, and that we will never again be the person we once were.

With this realization comes an important fork in the road. Yogi Berra said, "When you come to a fork in the road take it." One fork leads to living out our life thinking about the past, how good we used to be, and lamenting that we just can't do the things we used to. This fork inevitably leads to discouragement, isolation, and spending our remaining days within ourselves. The other fork leads to realistically but optimistically heading toward joyfully living out our life.

There are some key steps in taking the "joyful fork":

1. Be thankful for the life you have had and the blessings you have received. It's not only okay to look back, but it's helpful if it's with a healthy attitude.

2. Remind yourself that God has you here for a reason. Don't quit now.

3. Be comfortable with yourself—as you are now!

4. Start each day with a prayer similar to the well-known prayer, "God grant me the serenity to accept the things I cannot change, the courage

to change the things I can, and the wisdom to know the difference."

5. Focus on others, not yourself. It is crucial to shift our minds from dwelling on just our own issues and problems to how we can help others. It might only be in some small way, but the key is let your life become **not** all about you!

Every day of your life, there will be someone out there who needs the joy you can share. Perhaps it's someone very close to you. Find them. Bring them joy!

The joyful and happy older folks I know have discovered this simple notion: that life's not about them, but about others. It's interesting that not a single one of these friends who are focused on others are discouraged, lonely, isolated, or feeling worthless. They all have retained their self-respect. As it turns out, I am the only one that can cause me to lose my self-respect. It's the same with you—no one can take away your self-respect but yourself!

So, get out there and play as long as you can. Spike it if you can. If you can't spike, then set. If you can't set, then sit on the sideline and cheer. If you can't cheer, then pray for the players—and smile! After all, God is cheering for you, **dagnabbit!**

CHAPTER 6:
PURPOSE IN LIFE

═══════════════

OLD IS WHEN…You own a "smart-phone" but don't know how to turn it on.

I love having a purpose in life. I love having a reason to get out of bed each morning. I don't think I'm alone in this thought either. In fact, it seems to me that everyone, yes, every single one of my **joyfully** aging friends have this common thread—they have at least one purpose in their lives. They look forward to the next day, and the next. That's right, even while aging; look forward to the next day. Let's explore this "purpose notion."

Years ago when I watched the Miss America competition with my friends, we joked about the judges' questions to the contestants. When the top five were interviewed, the master of ceremonies would quite often ask, "What would you like to accomplish in life?" The most common answer **was to bring about world peace**. Well, good for them. I think if that is your goal, then good for you, but for most of us aging dudes and dudettes, our purposes are not so lofty. Most of us are focused on real-life purposes that we can accomplish in our lifetimes. We want to make a difference before it's too late!

I have a friend and neighbor in her late 70s who described herself as living in a cocoon for a year following the death of her husband. She now looks back and realizes that she was engaging in self-pity and not focused on anything but herself. She now maintains that happiness is a choice and seeks to spread joy to at least one person every day.

Yet another friend and neighbor in his 80s, also recently widowed, starts every day focusing on his friends and family. In general, he focuses on the positive side of their lives. He has kids and grandkids that are making poor choices in their lives, but my friend chooses to start his day thinking of something they might do well. He's not oblivious to their shortcomings, but by focusing on the positives, he's better equipped to really relate to them and help them. These positives are:

—Live life a day at a time

—Think on positive things

—Have a purpose(s) regarding something other than yourself

I know for me it's a matter of limiting the number of purposes I focus on at any one time. I'm extremely blessed in having good health, good "go-getter" energy, and lots of interests to pursue. The down side is that I sometimes find myself having so many things on my plate that I don't properly pursue any of them. So here's what works for me. At the start of each year I consider what my top three purposes are in life. That's right, I limit the number to three—then I write them down. Somehow, this seems to work. It forces me to prioritize, then by visibly looking at the list of three things I take a minute to consider them. Are these really the things that I want to spend my time and effort on this year? Sometimes opportunities come about during the years that affect my priorities, but here's the rule for me: If I add a purpose to my top three list, something has to drop from the list. For me, I can only have so many bouncing balls in the air at one time to do justice to my "purposes." I think God also puts before us opportunities to serve others and bring a little joy into their lives on a daily basis.

Now, here's the thing about some of us older Christians. Sometimes we are guilty of making our purposes so broad that they're almost meaningless. "To save the world" is almost like "to bring about world peace" in the sense that they are lofty, well-meaning, and wholly holy, but they give me no sense of real purpose. A purpose needs to be something I **can** accomplish. Give a thirsty person a drink of water, help a child with their studies, listen to a friend, take a granddaughter to dinner—the kinds of things Jesus encouraged us to do!

For some of us, the time we have left on this earth is getting short. It's time, then, to take stock of our purpose for being here and each day focus on how we can better fulfill these purposes. What a difference it can make to realize what we do matters and that we **can** make a difference. When you discover your purpose, TAKE JOY, **DAGNABBIT!**

CHAPTER 7:
TODAY IT IS
(Living life one day at a time)

═══════════════

OLD IS WHEN...The "little old lady" you are helping cross the street is your wife.

A really interesting statement comes from the writings of noted psychiatrist Dr. James C. Fisher. He says, "If you were to take the sum total of all authoritative articles ever written by the most qualified of psychologists and psychiatrists on the subject of mental hygiene, and if you were to have these unadulterated bits of pure scientific knowledge concisely expressed by the most capable of living poets, you would have an awkward and incomplete summation of the SERMON ON THE MOUNT. And it would suffer immeasurably through comparison."

Dr. Fisher continues, "For two thousand years the Christian world has been holding in its hands the complete answer to its restless and fruitless yearnings. Here...rests the blueprint for successful human life with optimum mental health and contentment."

WOW—and what did Jesus say in the Sermon on the Mount when summing up how to live a life of contentment? "Therefore, do not worry about tomorrow, for tomorrow will worry about itself. Each day has enough trouble of its own." Matthew 6:34

Several of the joyfully aging individuals that I've interviewed told me the same thing. In the words of LaVerne from her assisted living home, "I just do life a day at a time." She explained that she has now realized that today is all there is, and not to put off until tomorrow anything that needs to be said or done because tomorrow may not come for her. Similarly, she says she has managed to stop worrying about the future. She focuses on today. In her words, the purpose of life each day is "...to reach out to someone today in such a way that they would seek to know God."

This thread seems so consistent in the joyfully aging camp. It seems like one has to reach old age to comprehend what Jesus was saying (and some never get it). He wasn't suggesting that we live in a worry-free world where there are no future problems. He wasn't saying we should be ignorant and "willy-nilly" about the future. It's just that the future should not be our focus. We ought not to spend all our time and energy worrying about tomorrow or yesterday. It's about today, and should be only about today. Live in the moment!

———————

THE LAST DANCE—please allow me to share a personal note to illuminate the point. About 2 months before my wife Barb died of gastric cancer, we were preparing to attend a wedding which included dinner and dancing. Since it had been a while since we had danced we decided to practice beforehand. We put some music on and danced in the tiled kitchen area of our home that Barb and the contractor had recently beautifully remodeled. We later attended the wedding, but Barb was too ill for us to stay for the dinner and dancing. Here's my point—my last dance with my wife "Barbara Darlin'" of 58 years…was in our kitchen, and I'm afraid I didn't really cherish it at the time! I'm sure I was more focused on the dance, and how we might look on the dance floor later. You may say, "Yes, but you had no way of knowing that the kitchen dance would be your last," and that's exactly the point. We don't know when something to be cherished is happening for the last time. So cherish your life today—there may actually be **no** tomorrow.

Let me plead with you to cherish the moment—especially the moments with your mate. You might be sitting in church together and your wife holds your hand, or sitting together on the patio watching a hummingbird, or picking out a Christmas tree together. JUST PAUSE—AND CHERISH THE MOMENT!

Jesus was right-on about this one—It's TODAY, **dagnabbit!**

CHAPTER 8:
ALL RIGHT AT THE END

Old IS WHEN…Well, we just know, don't we?

I went to a movie called *The Best Exotic Marigold Hotel* recently where I heard a saying that sank in with me. The young actor from India said to his hotel guests— ***"Everything will be all right at the end. If things are not all right, then it is not yet the end."***

I like that!

In our journey through this little book together, we've learned a few things about some of the problems of aging and some things about **joyfully** aging in spite of the problems. But one thing seems crystal clear: Life is never going to be perfect—not in this life! But, as the saying describes—this is not yet the end!

Kay Warren says it well in her definition of **joy**, from the book *Choose Joy*, where she describes **joy**, in part, as:

THE QUIET CONFIDENCE THAT, ULTIMATELY, EVERYTHING IS GOING TO BE ALL RIGHT.

I think that's it—the quiet confidence that ultimately everything is going to be all right!

Even in death, the quiet confidence can still be a part of it if you let it. When my wife died in 2012, I confess it took me a while to rekindle my joy. But I took great solace and joy in the support of my family and friends, and within a couple of months I began to realize that I still had the quiet confidence that, ultimately, everything was going to be all right. I then again began sharing my joy. I still believed JOY is a choice, but I was finding it difficult to mesh joy with real sorrow. Then I realized—that's exactly what the examples of the joyfully aging that I've written about in this book are doing...BEING JOYFUL, EVEN IN SORROW. The sorrow is real, but I remain convinced that JOY is real as well.

So, let me summarize what I believe the most critically important things to remember and focus on if we are to age with joy. I've reduced the number to five. Since I'm writing to me (as well as to you) and I can never remember more than five things, here goes—DRUM ROLL, PLEASE!

Number 5—KEEP YOUR SELF-RESPECT. I'm not the man I once was—I'm just not. You may not be the person you once were either, but as we've discussed in this book, that's not what is really important. What counts is how we're doing in the things God says are important like the "fruit of the spirit." Namely, they are love, joy, peace, patience, kindness, goodness, faithfulness, gentleness, and self-control. Take stock of these nine areas of your life and compare each with how you were, say, 30 years ago. You know what you will likely find— that you're a lot closer to growing into the person God wants you to become than you could have imagined becoming years ago. Take JOY in knowing you are becoming what God wants you to be, and that's what matters. It's okay to like yourself, even love yourself, and retain your self-respect, **dagnabbit!**

Number 4—HAVE PURPOSE IN YOUR LIFE. As I've shared in this book, it seems to be a common thread of the joyfully aging to have real and meaningful purpose in our lives. We're not talking about bringing about world peace here unless that's what you (and Miss America) want to shoot for. We're talking about purpose that's attainable. Maybe it's helping the next-door widow with her chores, looking for someone at the grocery store who might need help paying for the grocery items, being a caregiver, or being a better grandparent. Focus on the purpose(s) in your life, **dagnabbit!**

NUMBER 3—MAINTAIN QUALITY RELATIONSHIPS. With both family and friends, recognize the value of relationships. They are sometimes harder to accomplish in old age, but well worth the effort. Cherish every relationship, work at it if need be, do your share in keeping it whole, and "for cryin' out loud," if you love someone—**tell** them! Relationships are a lot like life itself; they get harder. But they also get better if you let them, **dagnabbit!**

NUMBER 2—LIVE LIFE A DAY AT A TIME. It seems this is part of the distinctive joy of being in the Lord, to know where we're headed and simply do what we can today. The joyfully aging I know have figured out God was right about this one. Don't get all wrapped up in how everything might play out for the rest of your life, but focus on today. Even the adversities we face in old age don't seem like such a big deal if we tackle them a day at a time. Cherish the day, and do all you can to make it a great one, **dagnabbit!**

AND...NUMBER 1—**Finally: JUST GIVE JOY.** That's right, one of the great ironies we've discovered together is we don't set out to get joy, but to give joy. Then, by some strange and magnificent miracle, **we get joy ourselves from giving it!** Should this be the only thing you remember from this book, then our journey together has been a success. Be a "joy spreader." Focus on others and how you might bring a little joy into their lives. That's it, just give joy, and we'll all get it in return, **dagnabbit!**

Growing old can be the most meaningful and significant time of our entire lives. Let's not waste it in self-pity and self-indulgence. God still has us on this earth for a reason, and that reason could well be what we do today. Let's approach each day with the joy the Lord intended.

TAKE JOY IN GROWING OLD, DAGNABBIT!

EDGAR AND LEROY: THE CONCLUSION

═══════════════

"Well, I'll be," the usually grumpy old Leroy said to Edgar with a hint of a smile and a little twinkle in his moist eyes. "You know, Edgar, these common threads you describe in the joyfully aging are not all that complex and don't seem that hard to me."

"You're right, they're not that hard and I want to emphasize that you **are** qualified to take joy in life, especially in aging," Edgar replied. "An awful lot depends on making the choice to take joy, then going about living it day by day."

"Well," stated Leroy, "let's say I give this joy business a shot. What I think you said was that the top threads of aging with **joy** are:

- Keep my self-respect

- Have purpose in my life

- Maintain quality relationships

- Live my life a day at a time, and

- Just give joy

"Did I get it right?" asked Leroy.

"You nailed it. Perfect," Edgar replied.

"I'm excited to get started," Leroy said. "But first, something I want you to know— you bring me joy every day, and I love you, man. Now, where do I start?"

Edgar responded, **"I think you just did!"**

TAKE JOY IN GROWING OLD, DAGNABBIT!

CPSIA information can be obtained
at www.ICGtesting.com
Printed in the USA
FFOW04n1640040117
30984FF